HELP!
WHAT DO I DO NOW?

CARING FOR YOUR LOVED ONE WITH ALZHEIMER'S

HELP!
What Do I Do Now?

CARING FOR YOUR LOVED ONE WITH ALZHEIMER'S

Nancy Nicholson, LBSW

Help! What Do I Do Now?
Caring for Your Loved One with Alzheimer's

Lillie's Lovely Little Publishing Company
San Antonio, Texas
www.lillieammann.net
info@lillieammann.net

Editor: Lillie Ammann

Photo Credits
cover: Alexander Raths, Dreamstime.com
page 4: Yukchong Kwan, Dreamstime.com
page 18: Gemacanon, Dreamstime.com
page 21: Scott Griessel, Dreamstime.com
page 40: Yanik Chauvin, Dreamstime.com
page 46: Lisa F. Young, Dreamstime.com
page 55: Lisa F. Young, Dreamstime.com
page 61: Vladimir Voronin, Dreamstime.com
page 63: Lucian Coman, Dreamstime.com
page 69: Joy Fera,Dreamstime.com

ISBN 978-0-9665912-1-7

DEDICATION

To my beloved father, Harvey Nicholson, who was the first face of Alzheimer's I saw. Caring for him inspired my passion for working with the elderly, especially dementia patients.

To my beloved mother, Ann Nicholson, who was the first face of Alzheimer's caregiving I saw. Her constant devotion to my father throughout the progression of the disease inspired my appreciation for the love and commitment of caregivers.

ACKNOWLEDEGMENTS

Several people took the time to review the manuscript and share their valuable insights. Their input made this guide better, and for that I thank them. Any errors are mine alone.

Father Ed Morgan, Associate Rector of All Saints Anglican Church in San Antonio, who spent six years as a hospital chaplain in critical care areas where he worked with many Alzheimer's patients.

David Bowles, author of The Westward Sagas series of historical novels, whose cherished brother suffered with Alzheimer's.

Beverly Ellison, owner of Administrative Support Services, who has been caregiver for her mother with Alzheimer's for six years.

TABLE OF CONTENTS

PREFACE

This booklet began life as a school project. I had returned to college after a break of many years. During that break, I was one of the caregivers for my father, who had Alzheimer's disease (AD). He was diagnosed about twenty years ago, when the disease wasn't as well-known as it is now. Our family had never heard of Alzheimer's and had no idea what to expect or what to do. We learned a great deal as we cared for Dad for the last seven years of his life. Some of our education came from reading and from talking to doctors. Most of it, however, came from trial and error.

Caring for my father impacted me so profoundly that I decided to make a career of working with the elderly. I have worked in several capacities and went on to earn a degree in social work. My personal experience of caring for a loved one with this disease has been the most useful source of information for caregivers.

When I was assigned a project in college to create an informational pamphlet, Alzheimer's disease was the obvious topic for me. I wanted to help other families who were caring for loved ones with the disease. The project earned me an A and many compliments. My sister has encouraged me to make the information available to a wider audience, so now I have expanded the booklet to include more details as well as examples of how others have successfully handled specific situations.

Though the guide started as a class assignment, it has always been a labor of love. It is my hope that in these pages you find practical advice, encouragement, and hope.

INTRODUCTION

Alzheimer's disease (AD) affects not only the person diagnosed with the disease, but his family and friends as well. This booklet is intended to help you, the caregiver, deal with some of the challenges this disease presents. I've listed some common areas in which you might encounter obstacles and offered suggestions on how to handle them. I've also included some examples of how caregivers have dealt with specific issues. The scenarios are based on actual experiences but are composites of several different individuals and situations.

Please remember that Alzheimer's affects each person differently. You may not encounter all of the obstacles I've listed, and you may be presented with some that I haven't covered. Also keep in mind that different approaches work for different people. These tips come from my own experience, the experience of other caregivers, and ideas gathered from various resources, but you will have to find what works best for you and your loved one. Patience, humor, understanding, ingenuity, and flexibility are vital when caring for an Alzheimer's patient.

I have also included some tips on taking care of yourself. Caring for someone suffering from AD is a very demanding and stressful job. You cannot care for someone else if you do not first care for yourself.

There are many other aspects of caring for an Alzheimer's patient—such as legal or medical matters—I haven't covered. I did not include these because I wanted the focus of this booklet to be on the daily lives of AD patients and their caregivers. You may find the resources at the back of this booklet useful in getting the help you need with other important issues involved in caregiving. I hope the information and advice in this booklet will make your life just a little easier.

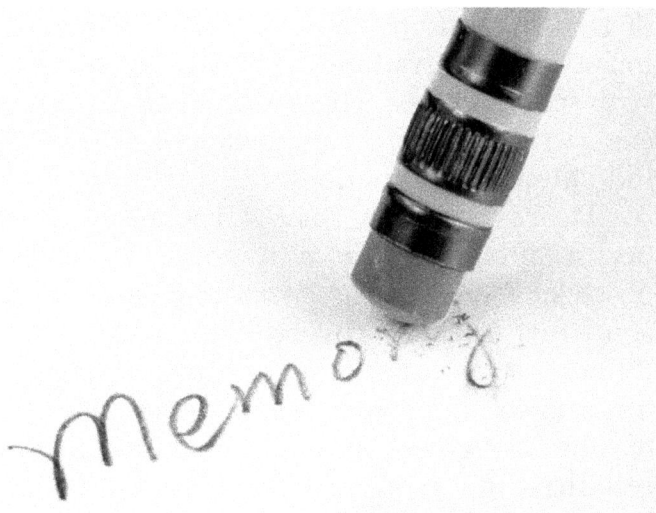

WHAT IS ALZHEIMER'S?

Significance of Alzheimer's

Alzheimer's is a progressive neurological disease that affects over 5 million Americans, and this number is expected to increase as the baby boomers age. AD is the most common type of dementia. The only way to definitely diagnose AD is through an autopsy. Most doctors diagnose the disease by the process of elimination. They test for other causes of the symptoms, and if all of those are eliminated, they make the diagnosis of Alzheimer's disease.

Alzheimer's is a brain disease, a type of dementia, like breast cancer is a type of cancer. Since Alzheimer's is a disease of the brain, it will impact all aspects of one's life—memory, cognition, judgment, communication, vision, personality, comprehension, walking, and the ability to perform routine tasks. Ultimately, the disease is fatal.

Alzheimer's affects not only the 5 million sufferers, but also their families and friends. Almost 11 million Americans spend billions of hours every year as unpaid caregivers for loved ones with AD. Caregiving can be stressful, time-consuming, and extremely difficult. This guide is designed to help make the task a little easier and less stressful.

Symptoms of Alzheimer's

Early symptoms of AD may be subtle and explained away as normal *forgetfulness*. After my father was diagnosed, we realized that some of his previous actions were symptoms of the disease. On one occasion, he drove to town to pick up my two nephews and came home without them. When Mom asked where they were, Dad said he had forgotten what he went to town for. Another time, my father, who always wore a tie to church, asked my mother to help him because he couldn't remember how to tie it. We thought Dad was forgetful, but we didn't recognize these incidents as symptoms of a disease until after he was diagnosed with Alzheimer's.

Memory Loss

AD patients first forget the latest things they've learned. They may forget a recent event or conversation yet remember in vivid detail their first day on their first job or their graduation from junior high. They may ask the same question repetitively because they don't remember they've asked before.

They tend to forget things in the reverse order that they learned them. Engineers may retain engineering knowledge, even though it is very complicated. However, they may forget early in the disease how to send email since they learned that much later in life. This is known as retrogenesis. There is some disagreement as to whether it exists, but I have observed it over and over through the years. For example, I have seen many bilingual AD patients lose the ability to speak in their second language and revert back to their native tongue.

Music and singing seem to be retained more frequently than other abilities. Music and verbal skills use different parts of the brain—the part of the brain required for speaking may be badly affected, but the part of the brain used for music may still be alert. Often, someone with Alzheimer's who has deteriorated to the point that they are nonverbal or speak only gibberish can sing along and remember all the words when they hear music, especially a favorite song or a cherished hymn.

People forget where they parked their cars at the mall and wonder if they have Alzheimer's. Forgetting something like where you parked your car is normal forgetfulness. People with Alzheimer's might find themselves at the mall, not know how they got there, and forget that they even have a car.

Changes in Cognition

AD patients are unable to learn new things—even if they are simple. What seems easy and natural to learn for most of us is complicated for the AD patient.

They can't make logical connections—if faced with a situation that is slightly different from their past experience, they can't figure out the similarities and adjust for the differences. For example, they can't figure out how to turn on a new TV because the on/off button is in a different position on the remote control.

They can no longer handle money. They may get confused and not pay the electric bill, then not understand why the power is shut off. They may order items they don't need from TV or Internet and not understand why the charges appear on their credit card statement. They can't balance their checkbook and may overdraw their account and not have any idea of where the money went. They may even give away money or other valuables to strangers.

Confusion

AD patients become confused and overwhelmed easily. Too much information tends to bewilder them. Too much stimulation overwhelms them. Often, they can focus on only one topic or activity at a time. Trying to keep track of two or more things at once is more than they can handle. When they become tired, they are more easily confused and anxious.

They tend to get lost even in familiar neighborhoods. They may put things in strange places, such as the car keys in the refrigerator, because they are confused.

Routine is very important to someone with Alzheimer's. Changes in schedule and surroundings and being in strange situations or around unfamiliar people can be very stressful. They may want everything in a specific place or tasks performed in a particular order.

In the early stages, they may need a reminder to do something, such as dress. As the disease progresses, they will need more instructions on how to complete the task, such as "Put on your shirt and your pants." In the later stages of the disease, you may need to tell them the first step and not move on to the next step until they have completed step one. Eventually, they will be unable to perform the task at all and will depend on you to do it for them.

Changes in Communication

Alzheimer's patients have problems in communicating—both in expressing themselves and in understanding what is said to them.

When speaking, they may lose their train of thought or have difficulty knowing the right word. What they say isn't necessarily what they mean.

They may not understand what is being said and consequently may answer inappropriately. If you have to repeat something they don't understand, they get confused if you say the same thing in different words. They think you are saying something totally different because their brain is still trying to process what you said originally.

Body language is very important. They may not be able to understand your words, but they recognize and respond to your tone of voice, position, and demeanor. If you get too close to them, lean over them, and speak loudly, they will probably become very agitated, regardless of what you say. On the other hand, if you smile, get at their level, and speak softly, they will probably respond positively, even if they don't understand your words.

Personality Changes

Often Alzheimer's patients become more childlike and innocent. They usually become more emotional, with emotions ranging from crying to anger to suspicion.

They lose their inhibitions, which can have both good and bad consequences. They may be willing to try things that they would never have done before. The introvert may come out of his shell. This often brings them great enjoyment.

> Dad was always friendly and pleasant, but he tended to be a homebody and didn't like to draw attention to himself. My sister, a

9

business owner, signed up for a seminar at sea. She could take guests for the cruise, and she invited me to go with her. When I told my parents about the upcoming trip, Dad asked, "Why didn't she invite us?" It had never occurred to either of us that Mom and Dad would want to go, but we were both glad to have them join us.

On the second day of the cruise, my folks said they were going to walk around the deck while my sister attended a seminar session and I went to a show. When we met up later for lunch, Mom announced, "Your father won the men's knobby knee contest." My sister and I looked at each other, then from my mother to my father. Dad had the cute little grin that we all loved. My sister and I thought Mom was joking, but they both assured us it was true.

Mom had become overtired when they were walking, and they looked for the first place they could find to sit down. The room they entered turned out to be an auditorium. A lady came up to Dad and invited him to enter the knobby knee contest. Dad went up on stage and let a bunch of strange ladies feel his knobby knees. He got a kick out of being declared the winner and being handed a little plastic trophy.

Later, after Dad's diagnosis, we realized he had been in the very early stage of AD and had lost his inhibitions. He had a good time being the center of attention, something he ordinarily avoided, and Mom, my sister, and I enjoyed his pleasure. My sister still has the little plastic trophy as a reminder of that fun vacation.

The loss of inhibitions can be positive, but on the other hand, patients may exhibit inappropriate behaviors or become very angry and verbally and/or physically aggressive.

They may become very needy and follow you everywhere. They want you with them all the time and become anxious if you are out of their sight. This may be because they are afraid of making a mistake or getting lost, and they feel safe with you.

It is very common for there to be a complete personality change. The father who wielded a heavy hand with his kids may become a sweet, gentle teddy bear. On the other hand, a prim and proper churchgoing mom may become angry, cold, and as foul-mouthed as any sailor. The personality change is often the most difficult for families to deal with and often causes the most chaos, pain, and embarrassment for them.

Changes in Social Interactions

One of the early symptoms of Alzheimer's is withdrawal from social activities. They may quit going to church or the civic club or stop socializing with friends and extended family. At this point, the AD patient recognizes that something is wrong and wants to avoid situations in which others will recognize the change. Loved ones may not yet notice other symptoms of AD and wonder why the individual is refusing to participate in normal activities.

Through the progression of the disease, relationships with loved ones change. The once-strong and independent father becomes the child. The man who was the head of the family has to depend on his wife to make simple decisions. The mother who taught her children by example has to be told to get dressed in the morning. Family members and friends often find the changes in the relationship hard to handle.

Many AD patients lose the ability to empathize with other people. They become so focused on their own needs that they seem to be selfish and uncaring about those around them. They are more concerned about their minor problems than about serious problems of their loved ones. They may sometimes be very loving and thoughtful when it does not inconvenience them. However, when they want something, they ignore the illness or injury of their caregivers and want the caregivers to respond to their wishes immediately. They act as if the world revolves around them.

Sometimes people with Alzheimer's remember things that happened in the past and forget everything since then. There may have been an estrangement from another family member that was later healed or an argument that was later resolved. The AD patient may forget the forgiveness and reconciliation and refuse to have anything to do with the other person, thinking they are still estranged.

Alzheimer's is a very isolating disease, both for the person who has it and for the family. AD affects the family in a different way from other serious diseases. While loved ones of someone who suffers with cancer or who has had a stroke are certainly greatly affected by the disease, the family of a person with AD has a more difficult time accepting help from others. The confusion, fear, anger, emotions, and behaviors of the Alzheimer's patient make it almost impossible for those unfamiliar with the disease to help.

Not only are the behaviors of the patient hard to deal with, but also until the very late stages, Alzheimer's patients don't look sick. People who don't know anything about the disease may think that the patients aren't ill but simply being difficult.

> Rita had never been a regular churchgoer, but she attended special services such as Easter and Christmas with her husband, Herb. Herb, on the other hand, rarely missed a service and served on numerous committees at church. Once Rita was diagnosed with Alzheimer's, Herb was unable to attend church on a regular basis. He never knew what Rita would do if left home alone. She might go for a walk and get lost or put something on the stove and forget about it.
>
> Members of the church offered to assist Herb so that he could again attend services. The women's group agreed to have members rotate Sundays in which one of them would stay with Rita while Herb attended church. Alice was the first to volunteer; she and her husband had known Rita and Herb for over 30 years. They had been a real source of comfort and strength for Alice when her husband fell ill and passed away several years before. Alice arrived at Rita's home 30 minutes before services were to start and saw Herb out the door, assuring him that everything would be fine.
>
> As soon as he left, Rita began asking when he would be back and why was he taking so long. Alice tried to reassure Rita and to distract her by suggesting that they bake some bread. Things seemed to be going

well once they started the bread project, but halfway through Alice turned around to see Rita adding more flour to the mixture. Alice asked Rita what she was doing, and Rita answered, "Making bread." Alice explained that they had already added the flour and Rita had just ruined the bread. Rita assured her that she could fix it by adding more water and promptly placed the mixture under the faucet and turned it on. The mixture became a soupy mess before Alice could grab the bowl from Rita's hand.

Rita stomped out of the room. Alice found her in the living room crying and saying, "When is Herb going to be home?" Alice didn't know what to do, and she, too, began to hope that Herb would return soon. Alice tried to clean up the mess before Herb got home, but he arrived before she had completed the task. He looked around the room, laid down his Bible, and said, "I see she gave you a run for your money." Alice tried to act as if the situation wasn't a big deal, but she left as soon as she could.

Alice and some of the other ladies tried to keep up their promise of helping, but they didn't know how to handle the angry outbursts, repetitive questions, and fragile emotional state of Rita. Gradually they began to say they were "too busy" or "had been missing too many services" or "my husband wants me in church with him." After a couple of months, Herb gave up the idea of attending church services and found a TV ministry that he could watch late at night when Rita was asleep.

Compensating

Even though they don't understand what is happening, Alzheimer's patients often recognize that something is wrong and try to hide it. They may cover it up with humor—when someone laughs at them because they've made a silly mistake, they laugh also as if they meant it as a joke.

They may be more likely to exhibit symptoms in environments in which they are comfortable. Caregivers often see behaviors that other people don't. Just as children often behave better in public than they do at home, patients may manifest more extreme behaviors when they are alone with their caregivers than they do when they around other people.

They may try to blame others for their forgetfulness or mistakes. They may deny that they did something or accuse someone else of being responsible. They may be very reluctant to take responsibility for their own actions. Many times they become angry out of frustration or embarrassment.

Susie loved plants. She went to the store to buy plants for some empty flowerpots on the patio. When she came home from the store with wind chimes but no plants, her husband Joe asked her where the plants were. Susie said he hadn't given her enough money to buy plants. However Joe knew that Susie had plenty of money in her purse and suspected that the wind chimes cost far more than the small plants she intended to buy.

He offered to help her hang the wind chimes, but she insisted she could do it herself. Joe watched as she methodically untied each chime and hung it over the back of a lawn chair. Joe asked, "How can you hear the chimes that way?" Susie answered, "Why would I want to hear them? They're to look at."

When she took the decorative ball that the chimes had been attached to and threw it to the dog, Joe started laughing and said, "What are you doing?"

Susie glanced at Joe and then started laughing herself. After a short pause, she said, "Oh, I'm just being silly."

Joe realized that his laughter had alerted Susie that she had done something wrong, but he could tell she didn't really know what it was.

Physical Changes

As Alzheimer's disease progresses, it affects walking, vision, and eating.

AD patients tend to walk in smaller steps and at a quicker pace. They may tend to bend forward or lean to one side.

They lose their peripheral vision, and they have problems with depth perception. They find patterns confusing. They may think the designs are bugs or debris rather than a part of the floor or tablecloth. Often, they think black places, such as black squares of tile on the floor, are holes and will step over or around the "holes" so they don't fall in.

They may eat all the time—possibly because they don't sit long enough to eat a complete meal or because they need more food because of the activity of pacing. They tend to crave sweets. They start to have difficulty feeding themselves and need help, and later they may need to be fed.

Stages of Alzheimer's Disease

While there are different thoughts about the stages of Alzheimer's, many experts agree that there are three stages. This is a guideline and not a hard and fast rule. There is not a point that stage one ends and stage two begins. There are overlaps between the stages, and patients do not progress on a steady line.

From time to time, they may seem to get better, then suddenly they get worse again. Even on a daily basis, the disease is variable. On some days, it may seem there is nothing wrong, but a short time later, the symptoms reappear, perhaps even stronger.

As the disease progresses and mental and physical functioning declines, your loved one will be moving on to the next stage. The amount of time that a person stays in each stage varies widely, and no one knows exactly why. Many factors can affect the progression of the disease.

Is the person on medication for AD? Are they in good physical health to begin with? I have seen over and over again that when a person suffers a physical setback it seems to jump start the speed of the progression of Alzheimer's. Anything from a cold to an infection to a heart attack seems to have an effect on AD. Usually as patients recover from the physical illness, their cognitive abilities improve also but often do not return to the same functioning as before the physical illness.

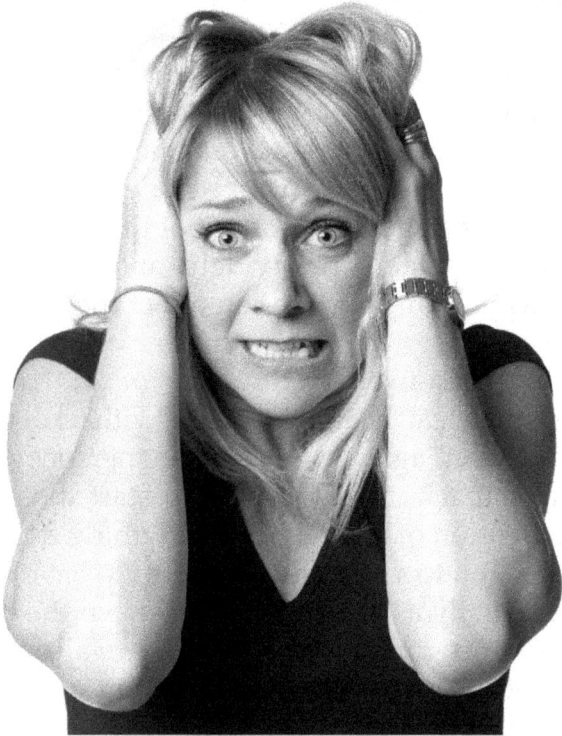

HOW DO I DEAL WITH ALZHEIMER'S?

Communication

Communication with an Alzheimer's patient can be very difficult and frustrating for both of you. At times he may not be able to express himself or may not be able to understand what you are trying to say. The following tips may enhance your communications with him.

- Never approach him from behind. Just think of how you are startled when someone walks up from behind you and touches you unexpectedly. Someone with Alzheimer's disease is already confused, frightened, and suspicious. Their reaction is often to fight back.
- Always let him see you when you're talking to him. If he cannot determine where the voice is coming from, he may become more confused or frightened. Position yourself in front of him and make eye contact when you speak.
- Be patient; trying to rush him will only make it more difficult for him to express himself.
- If he seems to be grasping for a word, try guessing what he is trying to say based on the context of the conversation.
- If he uses an inappropriate word, do not correct him. Verify your understanding by repeating what you think he meant. For example, if he said, "I went to the dog this morning," you may respond, "So you took the dog to the park this morning?"
- Don't become upset or argue with him.
- Gently touch his arm or shoulder, if necessary, to keep him focused on you.

- Address him by his name.
- Talk to him slowly and calmly.
- Use simple words and short sentences.
- Repeat yourself, if necessary, using the same words. Trying to rephrase what you have said may confuse him.
- Avoid raising your voice. Although you may simply be trying to help him hear and understand, he may think you are shouting at him. Even if he raises his voice, keep your voice calm and even.
- If he is unable to understand you, wait a while and try again.
- Ask questions that he can answer with "yes" or "no."
- Avoid saying things that he may take literally, such as "Jump into bed now."
- Realize that he can usually understand body language even when he cannot understand words. Be careful that you don't show frustration and anger in your body language.
- Learn to interpret your loved one's special communication.

Jermaine was in the middle stages of AD and had difficulty communicating consistently. He often told his sister/caregiver that he wished it would rain. His sister was puzzled by that statement and wondered why Jermaine would say such a thing. After a while his sister noticed Jermaine going toward the kitchen when he talked about wishing it would rain. Whenever his sister gave him something to drink, Jermaine gulped it down. The next time he said he wished it would rain, his sister gave him a glass of water. Jermaine drank it down and said, "I'm glad it rained." Jermaine was unable to correctly express himself, but his sister came to realize what he meant.

If your loved one does not understand you, try using gestures to enhance communication. If you want him to raise his leg, gently touch his leg to let him know what *leg* means. If he doesn't reply when you ask if he is thirsty, try motioning as if you were drinking from a glass. You can also have a picture board or book where you have pictures of common items and actions that the person with AD can point to.

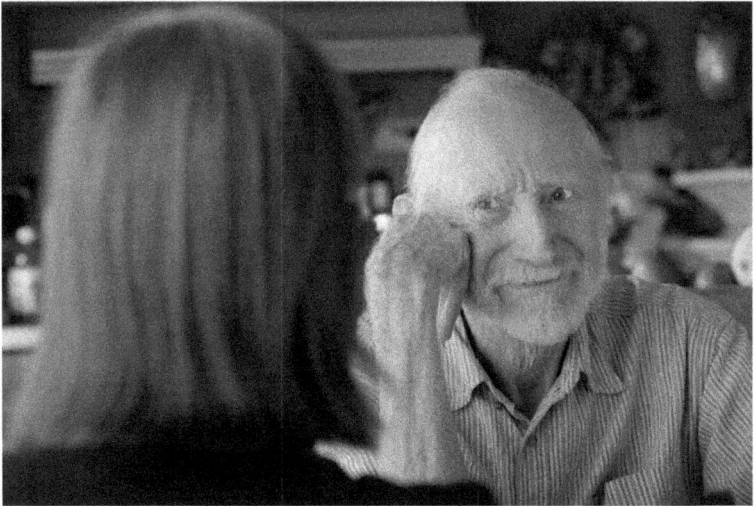

Behaviors

Disturbing or Inappropriate Behaviors

Alzheimer's patients may behave inappropriately and irrationally. However, there is a reason behind every behavior and what is irrational to us may seem perfectly rational to the AD patient.

The following are some common behaviors and ideas on how to handle them.

- He may flirt with everyone. This could be because of a loss of inhibitions or because in his mind, he is at a younger age when he was single and enjoyed flirting. Or he may mistake someone else for a younger version of his wife. Don't get upset. Try to distract him.

- He may become very clingy and want you within eyesight at all times, following you around like a little puppy. He knows that something is wrong, and he is afraid that he can't function on his own. He depends on you for a sense of security. Reassure him that you are close by. If you leave the room for a few minutes, let him know you are leaving and that you will return soon. If you move out of his eyesight, let him know where you are and assure him that you can hear him if he calls you. Give him frequent reassurance that you will not abandon him.

- He may ask repetitive questions—asking the same thing over and over again, sometimes almost constantly. It doesn't help the situation to tell him you've already answered the question—he doesn't remember even asking it. Sometimes you can give visual clues to remind him, such as a note that answers a question he asks frequently. Sometimes you can come up with creative solutions.

Eleanor's family took her purse with her Social Security card, driver's license, and other important documents home from the nursing home for safekeeping. Eleanor continually went to the nurses' station and asked everyone where her purse was. She became extremely agitated because she needed her driver's license, even though she hadn't driven for years. She wanted her comb and lipstick, also.

The staff was becoming annoyed at Eleanor's constantly searching for her purse. Then the social worker made a suggestion. She asked the family to bring Eleanor's purse with the documents along with another old purse and wallet on their next visit. She made copies of the documents, laminated them, and put them in the wallet. Then she put the wallet, along with a comb and tube of lipstick, in the old purse.

Eleanor was happy that she had her purse, her makeup, and her important documents with her at all times. The family was glad that they had the original documents safely stored at home, and the staff was happy that Eleanor no longer asked them dozens of times a day to help her find her purse.

A little imagination and flexibility made life easier for everyone.

- He may start undressing in public. This could be a result of physical discomfort. Do not get upset.

- Lead him to a private place and help him to redress.
- If this is a continuing problem, check to be sure that his clothes are comfortable and not too tight or too hot.
- Check to see if this may be an indication of needing to toilet.
- If you cannot determine his reason for removing his clothes, dress him in layers. Put an undershirt on him followed by a lightweight T-shirt and then a button-down shirt. You can dress him in boxers, followed by lightweight shorts, and then pants or warm ups. If he takes off the first or second layer, he will still be dressed.
- Try dressing him in a one-piece jump suit. This is more difficult to remove and may give you time to get to him before he completely disrobes.

- He may hallucinate and talk to people who are not there. This could be a side effect of medication, or it could be that he's misinterpreting what he is seeing, especially if he is looking at something with a pattern or design. Don't argue with him. Accept this as part of the disease.

Dad was very agitated, and I noticed that he continuously walked over to the wall, leaned over, and appeared to brush something off onto the floor. After several minutes of this, I walked over and asked him what he was doing. He looked at me and said "I'm killing these roaches. They're crawling all over the wall." I reassured him and tried to convince him that there were no roaches. All I accomplished was to agitate my dad even more and have him accuse me of trying to make him think he was crazy. Finally I went to the kitchen and retrieved the roach spray from under the sink. I went back to the living room and offered to help my dad with the roach problem. For the next couple of minutes I sprayed the wall as he pointed out the roaches. Together we took care of the problem. My dad was satisfied that the roaches were gone, and I was glad that his agitation was gone.

- He may accuse you or other family members of stealing, lying, or trying to hurt him. If he's misplaced something, he may be convinced that it was stolen and since you were the only person around, it had to be you. He may not remember something you've told him, and he thinks you're lying when you tell him now. Paranoia is part of the disease, and if he's afraid of something, he may blame you for the problem. Do not take this personally. Be reassuring and try to distract him.

It had become increasingly more difficult to get Dad to take his medications. Now it was to the point that he was getting angry. He would state, "I know what you are doing. You're trying to poison me." The look in his eyes made me want to cry. I thought, How must he feel if he thinks that his own family is trying to poison him?

- He may pay the wrong amount for things he buys or walk out of the store with items he hasn't paid for. He is confused about money or forgets that he has to pay for items he buys. If possible, go to stores where the people know you. Explain the situation beforehand and make arrangements for you to pay for the items or return them later. Have him carry a card that states he is memory impaired and that includes information on how to contact you.

- A person with Alzheimer's often becomes more amorous and desiring of sexual contact. He has lost his inhibitions, and in his mind, he is at a younger age. This may be handled differently depending on a variety of factors: Does the patient have a partner who can limit sexual activities to appropriate times and places? Is the individual living in a nursing home or other facility with established policies? Is the person making unwanted sexual advances to others? You (and/or the facility where your loved one lives) will have to decide how to handle this situation, but you need to be aware that it can become a problem.

Sometimes the actions of a person with Alzheimer's may be misinterpreted. Often they want to hold someone's hand or lie in bed with them simply for the comfort and security it brings.

Physical/Verbal Aggression

Many people with Alzheimer's disease exhibit physical and/or verbal aggression toward others. It is important to try to determine what causes the behavior. There is always a reason for someone to act the way that they do. It may not be a logical reason, but there is a reason behind every behavior. Determining the root of the behavior can help you find ways of preventing or alleviating it.

Sometimes the person is frightened and does not understand what is happening. A woman with AD may no longer recognize her husband. When he tries to bathe her, she may think that a strange man is attacking her and trying to hurt her. She may scream, scratch, hit, and kick at him.

Someone who can no longer communicate with words may use force to get her point across.

Stanley was at the point in the progression of his Alzheimer's that he no longer was able to communicate verbally. Although from time to time he would utter sounds, no one could understand any actual words. He was very protective of his room and did not like anyone to go there.

One morning when his daughter Daisy went into his room to change the sheets on his bed, he walked up behind her, grabbed her, and started pulling her. She was frightened and jerked away from his grasp. Stanley got in front of her and began pushing her, causing her to lose her balance and fall.

His wife Beth rushed in and helped Daisy to her feet, appalled at Stanley's actions. She had never seen him display physical aggression before. Once Daisy was on her feet, she and Beth quickly exited the room, followed by Stanley. He looked back at the room, closed the door behind him, and then calmly walked over to the couch and sat down.

The women discussed the incident and realized that Stanley simply did not want anyone in his room. Since he could not use words to communicate, he made his point the only way he knew how. His intent was not to harm anyone—but simply to get them to leave his space alone.

If your loved one does become verbally or physically aggressive, remember to stay calm. Always approach from the front and don't invade her space. Keep your voice friendly and your body language non-threatening. She may not understand your words but can interpret your body language. The anger often stems from frustration. She realizes that she is not capable of doing things that she is used to doing, and she strikes out. Anger can also come from fear or embarrassment. Whatever the cause, try to remember that it is not personal and not intentional. Do not try to physically restrain her as this will more likely cause her to fight even more. If she is not in danger of hurting herself, simply walk away and let her calm down.

My father had shown symptoms of Alzheimer's that we didn't recognize. However, after he had a heart attack, he went from mild to severe immediately. He had been sedated in the small-town hospital where he was first taken and was still under sedation after he was airlifted to a hospital in the nearest city and admitted to a private room. My sister and niece were sitting with him, and the staff at the hospital told them not to let him get out of bed if he woke up.

When he awakened, Dad said he needed to go to the bathroom. Fearing that he could cause serious damage by getting up, my sister hurried to get a nurse. The male nurse entered the room just after Dad stood up by the side of the bed with his back to the door. The nurse came into the room, reached across the bed, grabbed Dad's shoulders from behind, and sat him down on the bed. Dad came out fighting. The nurse called for help, and about eight nurses and aides showed up to restrain him. Thinking they were doing the right thing, my sister and niece helped hold him down. Everyone was amazed that a man who had just had a heart attack a few hours earlier could be so strong. My sister and niece had bruises for weeks from where Dad had hit them in the struggle. Finally the whole group held Dad down while nurses tied him up with restraints.

Tears still come into my sister's eyes when she remembers this incident. This was the first serious episode with Dad's AD, and family members simply followed the instructions of the medical staff. However, after it was over, they realized that the whole situation could have been avoided if Dad had simply been allowed to walk to the bathroom. If the nurse had approached him from the front, the situation might have been avoided and would certainly have been less serious.

Dad woke up in a strange room with no idea of what had happened to him. When he was grabbed from behind, he thought he was being attacked and fought to defend himself. He wasn't intentionally being physically aggressive—he was acting defensively.

If only our family and the medical staff had known to just walk away, this whole painful episode would never have happened.

Sundowning

A large percentage of Alzheimer's patients engage in a behavior called *sundowning,* which usually occurs in the evening—the time that the sun goes down. Although there has been a lot of speculation, the reason for this is unknown. One theory is that sundowning is connected to the shadows that are often seen at this time of day. Patients may exhibit an increase in restlessness, confusion, disorientation, and anxiety at this time of day.

Following are some common behaviors associated with sundowning and tips that may help reduce them.

- If he constantly paces, try taking him for a walk or providing activities that will give him physical exercise.
- Keep noise to a minimum. A noisy environment may add to his agitation.
- If he insists that he has to go to the store or to someone's house, tell him that you called and the store is closed or the people are not home.
- A glass of warm milk may help to calm him down.
- Allow him to walk as long as he is in a safe environment.

Every evening, Booker started pacing and walked and walked and walked. He would often go to the front door and try to leave. When asked where he was going, he couldn't answer. His son Dauntay tried locking the door with the key so Booker couldn't get out to the busy street in front of the house. However, when he couldn't get the door open, Booker became very agitated and verbally abusive to his son. If Dauntay tried to stand in front of the door to keep his father from exiting, Booker hit and slapped Dauntay.

One day Booker got outside, and in desperation, Dauntay knocked on the door from inside. Booker opened the door. Dauntay smiled at his father and said, "I'm so glad you're here. Please come in and visit." Booker came back inside the house as if he were coming to visit.

He sat down and Dauntay showed him some family scrapbooks. After a few minutes, Booker was ready to leave again. This time, Dauntay let him leave and again knocked on the door and invited him back in.

Dauntay did this night after night. Although it didn't keep his father from leaving several times each evening, it was easy to get Booker back into the house and calm for a few minutes.

Activities of Daily Living

Hygiene

A person with Alzheimer's may not consider hygiene to be important. You may have to remind him to bathe or brush his teeth. He may not shave for a week or more, and he may allow his hair to grow and become disheveled. As the disease progresses, it may become necessary for you to assist him or to perform these duties for him.

The following suggestions may make the process of bathing easier and safer.
- Install grab bars and adhesive anti-slip strips in the tub or shower, if possible.
- Use a hand-held shower head to make it much easier to assist him with his shower.
- Provide a shower/bath stool, available at medical supply stores and drugstores, so he can sit.

A little preparation beforehand may make the process go more smoothly:
- Gather everything you will need and put it within easy reach. You do not want to leave him alone in the shower or tub to get something you need.
- Be sure that the bathroom is warm before starting a bath or shower. Elderly people are often cold.
- Check the water temperature to make sure it's comfortable. It may reassure him if he checks the water also.
- Don't force him to shower or bathe if he seems afraid of the water. It is not necessary for him

to have a bath every day. He might let you give him a sponge bath if he won't get into the water.

- Be very gentle when bathing him because skin tears and bruises easily on older persons.
- Allow and encourage him to perform as much of the bathing process as possible.

Douglas resisted showering every day. No matter what his wife Dee tried, the process of showering was a traumatic one for both of them. On a friend's suggestion Dee tried having Douglas bathe instead of shower, but the results were no better. In fact, Douglas seemed terrified of stepping into the tub full of water.

The end result was that Douglas fought with his wife—even hitting and kicking her— every day when she tried to get him in the shower. Finally, Dee resorted to giving him a bed bath with very warm water and a washcloth, two or three times per week.

Dee had to accept the fact that this was the best that it was going to be and understand that at this point there was no reason to try to force Douglas to shower daily. She actually enjoyed the time that she spent with him during the bed bath instead of dreading the shower battle and becoming exhausted during the process. She could now relax and talk to Douglas during the bathing process, and he was much less agitated every morning.

She only went through the struggle of having him shower for doctor's appointments or special occasions. While this wasn't what she would prefer, she realized that many battles lay ahead and there were others that were more important.

Dressing

As the disease progresses, dressing may become more of a challenge for the Alzheimer's patient.

- Allow her to make choices about what she wears but limit her choices. Hold up two articles of clothing and ask, "Would you like to wear this or this?"
- If she wants to wear a checkered shirt with striped pants, let her. It's not the end of the world.
- Make it easy with button-down shirts or dresses that button up the front as it may become difficult for her to bend her arm or to follow simple instructions.
- Be sure that the clothes are comfortable and not too tight.
- If she has a favorite outfit, buy a duplicate, if possible, so she can wear one while you launder the other.
- Be sure that she wears safe shoes. House shoes that can slip off may cause her to trip.
- Dress her in shoes with Velcro closures. She may not stay still long enough to tie shoestrings securely, and she may trip if they become untied.
- If she can dress herself but has difficulty with buttons, zippers, etc., give her garments with Velcro fasteners, unless she undresses at inappropriate times.

Jose was a rugged cowboy who had worn jeans and boots his whole life. As he became more affected by AD, his caregiver suggested to his wife Maria that she buy him warm-ups and stretch shorts to wear. The caregiver also suggested that tennis shoes might be safer for him to wear instead of his house shoes. He had not worn boots in several months much to the dismay of Maria. The suggestion appalled Maria—Jose had never worn anything except jeans. And tennis shoes? Jose would never wear tennis shoes!

Several weeks later, Jose's caregiver was gone for ten days to visit out-of-state relatives. During that time Jose and Maria's children came to help out when they could, but more responsibility for caring for Jose fell on Maria. After several days of struggling for thirty minutes or more to get a pair of jeans on her husband, she asked their daughter Contessa to pick up a pair of warm-ups for Jose. The next morning, the warm-ups made the task of getting Jose dressed much easier and quicker.

Maria came to realize that Jose was no longer her rugged cowboy, and there was no reason to make his and her life more difficult by insisting that he wear what he always had. Although it hurt her to make this sacrifice since it was just one more reminder that her husband was slipping away, she realized that it was not only easier on her (and the caregiver), but it was also less stressful for Jose. Shortly afterward she purchased him a new wardrobe of warm-ups and even tennis shoes.

Toileting

Maintaining his dignity while helping with toileting is difficult but important. Some of the following tips may be helpful.

- Do what you can to keep him from becoming embarrassed or self-conscious. Allow him to hold a towel in front of himself if he wants to.
- If he becomes incontinent, inform his doctor and have him checked. This can sometimes be caused by an infection.
- If he is incontinent, treat the problem matter-of-factly and don't embarrass him.
- Ask him every couple of hours if he needs to go to the bathroom or take him if necessary. He may forget where the bathroom is or simply forget to go.
- Do not withhold liquids. Dehydration can be a serious problem.
- Treat him with respect and dignity when helping him with toileting or changing his diapers if he no longer has control.
- Limit his intake of caffeine (coffee, tea, colas, etc.). Caffeine may stimulate the bladder and contribute to incontinence.
- If he has a hard time urinating, turn on water in the sink. Running water may help him go.
- It may be easier for him to sit rather than stand to urinate.

Eating

Depending on the stage the patient is in, she will have different problems with eating. I've listed the tips that might be most helpful through the progression of the disease.

- In the early stages she may want to eat constantly. In that case, try the following:
  - Remove unnecessary items from the table. She may try to eat flowers or artificial fruit.
  - Fix several small meals a day instead of three larger ones.
  - Have healthy snacks—such as fruit, pretzels, granola bars, chicken fingers, and carrot sticks—available.
  - Remove plates and food from the table immediately after the meal so she will not continue to eat.
  - If she tries to eat from other people's plates, gently redirect her to her own plate.
  - Let her use a bowl instead of a plate and a spoon instead of a fork if she finds it easier.
  - Place a washcloth under the bowl to keep it from sliding.
  - Avoid using a tablecloth or placemats with a lot of design. This may confuse her. Solid colors are best.

- In later stages it may become difficult to get her to eat anything. It may also become more difficult for her to use utensils and to feed herself. In that case, try the following:
  - Do not present too many food choices, which may cause her confusion and frustration.
  - Fix her favorite foods often.
  - Be patient and let her eat slowly.
  - Many Alzheimer's patients like sweets, so try dabbing a small amount of honey on meat or mixing a little jelly with her vegetables, rice, or noodles.

- Make a milkshake out of Boost, Ensure, or any other brand of nutritional supplement drink.
- Be sure that her food is cut into small pieces.
- Let her drink from a baby's sipping cup or use bendable straws.
- Give her plenty of liquids to keep her hydrated. Water, fruit juices, and sports drinks, such as Gatorade, are best.
- Restrict caffeine; it stimulates the bladder and may actually contribute to dehydration.
- Provide finger foods such as fruit, pretzels, or carrot sticks.
- Avoid peanut butter, bananas, and any sticky food that may be difficult for her to eat and may cause her distress if it gets on her.

- As the disease progresses, it may become more difficult for her to eat. At this point you will probably have to feed her. The following may be helpful.
  - Sit in front of her when feeding her.
  - Puree her food or try baby food.
  - Prepare easy-to-eat foods such as Jell-O, mashed potatoes, and oatmeal.
  - Feed her small bites, allowing plenty of time between them.
  - Apply light pressure to her lips to encourage her to open her mouth.
  - Give her liquids often, after every couple of bites.
  - Be sure liquids are at room temperature.
  - To prevent choking, try using thicker liquids such as apricot juice or milkshakes.

You can also thicken other liquids with Thick-it (available in most drugstores) or Knox Gelatin.

- Verbally instruct her to chew, or if necessary, demonstrate.
- Remind her to swallow.
- Gently stroke her throat to help her swallow.
- If she is not eating, is having problems chewing, or chokes often, consult with her doctor.
- Never force her to eat.

Berta was no longer able to feed herself. A provider did the cleaning and cooked lunch and dinner. However her husband, Fritz, liked to fix her breakfast. Oatmeal had always been one of Berta's favorite foods, and it was simple enough for Fritz to prepare.

He always carried on a monologue as he fed Berta, who spoke only a few words that usually didn't make any sense. One morning, as he spooned oatmeal into her mouth, he asked, "Is the oatmeal good, sweetheart?"

A few seconds later, Berta said clearly and distinctly, "Not really, but that's all you feed me."

Fritz had a good laugh and a warm glow to realize that Berta was still there even if she couldn't communicate. "Tomorrow," he said, "I'll fix you scrambled eggs."

At some point she may not be able to eat at all, and you may be faced with considering the placement of a feeding tube. Ask your doctor questions to be sure that you understand the advantages and disadvantages of a feeding tube. When a person is near death, their body no longer requires nutrition so they naturally lose the desire to eat. Being fed through a tube provides nutrition but does not provide the pleasure and satisfaction of eating normally. You will need to determine whether a feeding tube will provide any benefit for your loved one.

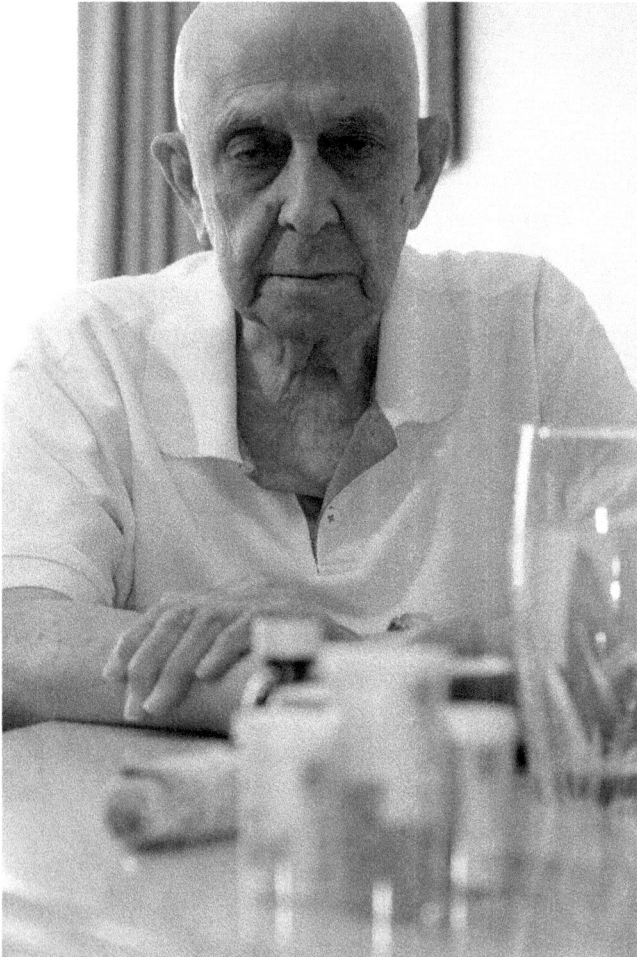

Administering Medications

It may become necessary for you to monitor his medications, and later on you may have to administer them to him. ALWAYS check with your doctor before changing anything to do with medicines. Some medications cannot be crushed; some must be taken with food; and some have other restrictions. You must ensure that you are administering medicines in a safe manner.

- Be sure that he takes his medication at the proper time.
- Monitor him to ensure that he swallows the pills.
- Familiarize yourself with the medications he takes and what each is for.
- Gently stroke his throat if needed to help him swallow his pills.
- Don't force him if he refuses to take his pills or accuses you of trying to poison him.
- Ask his doctor which pills can be crushed and put into applesauce or oatmeal if he is afraid to take them.
- If he won't take his medicine, wait awhile and try giving him the pills later.
- Discuss with his doctor the consequences of skipping each medication. Let her know of the difficulty he is having taking it. Maybe she can prescribe an easier form to take. Find out which ones can be skipped if necessary.
- Consider talking with his doctor about stopping some of the medications altogether. Is the medicine for high cholesterol really necessary at this point?
- If he is unable to give himself insulin shots, try having him hold something for you and then offer to give him the shot since his hands are full.

Safety

Safety of both the patient and the caregiver is a major concern for any person caring for an Alzheimer's patient.

Following are some suggestions on providing a safe environment for the patient.

- Keep all sharp objects, such as knives, scissors, and razors, locked away.
- Store medications, cleaning supplies, and chemicals where she cannot get to them.
- Ensure that there is adequate lighting in the home; sometimes eyesight deteriorates and it is harder to see in darker lighting.
- Keep matches and lighters in a safe place.
- Be sure that there are no loose rugs that she can trip on.
- If food is cooking on the stove or in the oven unattended, keep the door to the kitchen secured so that she can't accidentally wander in and burn herself.
- Lock doors to the outside or unsafe areas of the house, such as steep stairs. Either use a key or place a latch above eye level.
- Place childproof doorknob safety covers on doors to rooms that are not safe for her to enter alone.
- Simplify furniture arrangement and avoid clutter.
- Be sure to keep the house and furniture well-maintained to avoid danger from broken railings or unstable furniture.
- Install childproof locks for cabinets and closets.
- Remove knobs from the stove and oven, if necessary, to keep her from turning them on.

- At some point, you will probably have to determine that it is no longer safe for her to drive. The patient will likely be convinced that she is still an excellent driver. Giving up driving is a major issue, and it will be difficult for her to accept that she can no longer drive. However, for her safety as well as others on the road, it may become essential to keep her from doing so.

Suggestions for the safety of the caregiver follow.

- There may be danger to the caregiver because the AD patient may not recognize their family member and think he is an intruder. Avoid surprising them and make them aware of your presence and identity when you enter the house or the room.
- If the patient has weapons, such as guns or knives, the weapons should be removed or made inoperable (such as hiding the ammunition for guns).
- Don't fight or restrain the patient unless essential for safety. Walk away if the patient is kicking and fighting and give him space and time to calm down.

When You Can No Longer Manage

Alzheimer's progress at different rates for each individual. Although one study showed that, on average, death occurs from one to six years after diagnosis, many people live with AD for eight to twelve years and some for many more. As the disease progresses, the patient requires more and more care.

At first, your loved one may need only reminders. Then you have to deal with behaviors and assist with dressing and toileting. Eventually, caregiving will become a 24-hour, seven-days-a-week job. The AD patient will have times that she sleeps very little and wanders constantly. You must be vigilant to keep her safe. She may wander out at night or leave the stove on unattended. No one can keep up that pace for very long.

If you are lucky, you have other people who can help on a regular basis. But the reality is that most of your relatives and friends have families, jobs, and other responsibilities of their own. They may be able to help at times, but the majority if the caregiving is up to you. Don't feel guilty about asking for help.

You have several options to consider. Some organizations, such as the department of aging and disability services in your county or state and some local chapters of the Alzheimer's Association or AD support groups, have programs that provide respite care for AD caregivers. Usually the time is limited but flexible. It can be used for a few hours at a time throughout the month or used all at once for a day or two of rest. Nursing homes also have respite care where your loved one can stay anywhere from a couple of days to several months.

There may come a time that you will need to consider assisted living or nursing home placement for your loved one. Can you really provide the care that she needs and deserve all on your own? You may have health issues of your own; even if you are healthy, the stress of caregiving can become overwhelming. The patient may need skilled nursing care that you simply aren't qualified to provide.

In the early stages of the disease, when the patient just needs reminders and cues, assisted living might be the right choice. Most assisted living homes can help with the administration of medications and provide transportation and housekeeping services. However, they do not offer assistance with activities of daily living.

As time goes on, your loved one will need more assistance. At some point, it is likely that you will have to dress and feed the patient. She will be incontinent and display bizarre behaviors. The toll on you is both physical and emotional. If you become overwhelmed, you are more likely to be less patient and understanding, and you may even strike out at your loved one. While no one likes the idea of having a loved one in a nursing home, it may be the place where she can get the best care.

Just because she is in a nursing home doesn't mean that you don't love her. You can usually be at the home most of the day, and you can actually enjoy the time together because you aren't the one making her take her medicine or do other things she doesn't like. You can still help care for her, but you do not have the total responsibility. You are still her caregiver, ensuring she is receiving all the assistance and medical care that she needs.

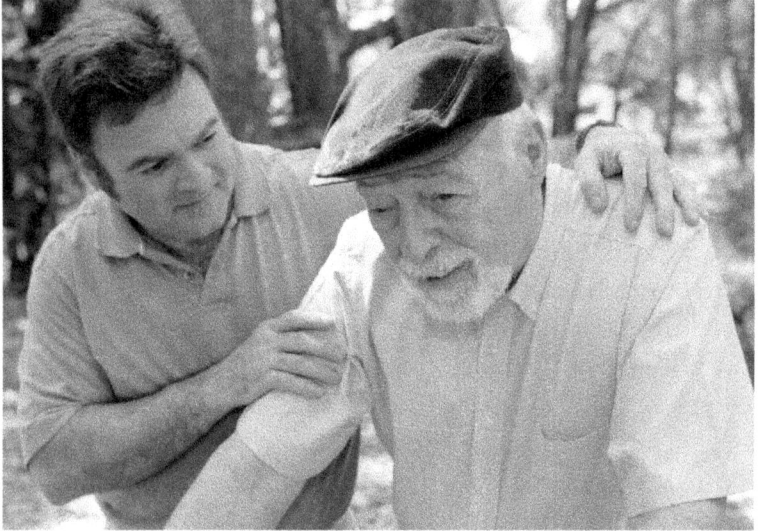

HOW DO I MAKE THE BEST OF THIS?

Choose Your Battles

As a caregiver for an Alzheimer's patient, you will face many challenges. In order to maintain your sanity, you will have to determine what is essential and what can be ignored.

In any situation, ask yourself, "How important is this battle?" If the patient's safety is involved, you must fight the battle. If the behavior is annoying or inconvenient or makes you feel uncomfortable, but doesn't cause any real harm, it may be better to give in and ignore it.

> LaToya didn't use sweetener in her coffee, but she collected packets of artificial sweetener everywhere she went. At the coffee hour after the service at her church, she went through the bowl of sweetener by the coffeepot, picked out all the pink packets, and stuffed them in her purse. When her family took her out to eat for a special occasion, she emptied the container on the table and asked the waitress for more "pink sugar." By the time they left the restaurant, she could hardly close her purse because it was so full of little pink packages of artificial sweetener.
>
> Her sisters were appalled at this behavior and tried to convince LaToya not to "steal the sweetener." When their appeals failed to stop the behavior, they started searching her purse

before they left the church fellowship hall or the restaurant and returning the sweetener packets to the containers. LaToya became very agitated whenever they did this, and she created a scene that embarrassed her sisters even more than the original act of taking all the sweetener had.

When her sisters asked her why she took the pink packets of sweetener, all LaToya would say was, "I need them." After many months, great embarrassment, and much frustration, LaToya's sisters decided there was no real harm in her hoarding packets of sweetener. Although they found it embarrassing, resisting it only made the situation worse. They vowed to ignore the behavior and even started bringing home packets of "pink sugar" whenever they went somewhere without her. She would get excited when her sisters gave her the little packages, and they enjoyed seeing her take such delight in such a simple thing.

Her sisters talked to the hostess of the church coffee hour and to the waitress at LaToya's favorite restaurant. Each agreed to put only a few packets of the sweetener on the table at a time. If LaToya asked for more "pink sugar," they simply said they were out. LaToya was satisfied with that answer.

Although this solution did not stop LaToya's behavior of picking up the packets of sweetener and putting them in her purse, it decreased the number of packets she accumulated and reduced her sister's embarrassment.

Sometimes you can make compromises. If the patient wants to eat only sweets, put more meat and vegetables on her plate with just a little something sweet. She can eat all the sweet food and only a small percentage of the rest but still end up eating more meat and vegetables and less sweets than she realizes. At some point, you may give her only sweets or whatever she wants because a balanced diet is less important than her enjoying what she likes during the latter stage of her life.

Although you may want to be completely honest with your loved one, sometimes "therapeutic lying" is the best approach. If she wants to give all her savings to a political candidate, simply tell her you have made the donation for her. If necessary, write out a check and show it to her with the promise to send it off, then tear it up and throw it away. Protecting her welfare while avoiding causing her distress is more important than absolute honesty.

Remember to keep answers simple. If she asks you where you're going and when you'll be back, there's no need to tell her that you're going to go to the grocery store for milk and juice and then to the meat market for a steak. You're also going to drop off a package at the post office and visit Aunt Ellen in the hospital. Simply reply, "I need to do a few errands, and I should be back by six."

A Comfortable Environment and Gentle Cues

The environment that your loved one with AD lives in can have an impact on her behavior. There should be good lighting and open spaces for her to walk without tripping. Solid colors on the walls, floor, and furniture are better than patterns and designs, which can confuse the patient.

Pictures of family members and your loved one when they were younger can be very helpful. Since she is regressing in time she may be more likely to recognize family members in pictures when they were younger. Music that she enjoyed in her teens and early adulthood may bring back good memories and help calm her. Favorite possessions—familiar room decorations or things she may have collected or enjoyed as a hobby—can make her environment more comfortable and pleasing for her. A glider rocker offers the movement of walking and may help cut down on wandering as well as bring her comfort.

You can use notes or cards to provide gentle reminders to your loved one.

> Since being diagnosed with AD, Enedelia had become used to having her husband Jaime with her all the time. On the rare occasions when he went to a doctor's appointment for himself or ran an errand alone, Enedelia would become agitated and frightened at being home by herself, even for only a short time. When Jaime returned, she would ask him, "Where have you been? Why did you go off and leave me?"

After this happened a number of times, Jaime started leaving notes for Enedelia. Since she wandered throughout the house, he left notes in every room in the place she was most likely to see them. In simple words Enedelia could understand, the note explained where Jaime was, when he would be home, and how to reach him. "I went to the post office. I'll be home at 11:00 AM. If you need me, pick up the phone receiver and punch 1. That will call my cell phone. Love, Jaime."

Enedelia never acknowledged seeing the notes, but each time Jaime left, she gathered all the notes up in a stack on the table beside her favorite chair. Occasionally she would call his cell phone and ask him when he was coming home, but hearing his voice reassured her and she no longer became agitated and frightened every time she was left alone.

You can use a similar technique to remind your loved one of where she is and what she is doing. Before you leave the house, give her a card to hold in her hand—"We're going to see Dr. Jones for your heart checkup" or "We're on our way to the grocery store." When she forgets, she can re-read the card rather than asking you every five minutes where you're going.

Use pictures of you, other family members and friends, and your loved one at various stages of life to help her recognize the people. If she becomes confused about who you are, you can show her photos of yourself when you were younger. Your mother is more apt to recognize you as a young child; your wife is more likely to recognize you as the young man she married. She may not even recognize herself in a mirror, but she may know that picture from forty or fifty years ago is her. She still sees herself as that beautiful young woman.

In her mind, Rosa was years younger. She didn't recognize herself in a mirror, but she did recognize her clothes. She would become very agitated when she looked in the mirror. She would shake her fist and shout, "Why are wearing my clothes? That's my favorite outfit. How did you steal it from me?"

Her husband, Carlos, tried to convince her that the woman in the mirror was herself and that no one was stealing her clothes. However, the problem got worse and worse until one day, Rosa doubled up her fist and tried to hit the "thief," slamming her fist into the mirror and breaking it.

After he cleaned and bandaged the cuts on Rosa's hand, Carlos went through the house and removed all the mirrors. Rosa never missed them, and she never again thought someone was stealing her clothes.

Telling Others

Your loved one may not want to admit anything is wrong, and she probably wouldn't appreciate your telling other people she has Alzheimer's disease. However, sometimes problems can be averted if others know about the patient's condition.

Any time the person with AD is receiving medical treatment, the medical providers need to be aware of the patient's condition. Even if your loved one is having an eye exam or routine dental work, AD can cause her to act in inappropriate or bizarre ways. You can discreetly inform the optometrist's or dentist's staff when you make the appointment. As the disease progresses, you may need to accompany the patient into the exam room, both to facilitate communication between the patient and the medical professional and to reassure your loved one that she is safe and that you caring for her and ensuring she is receiving appropriate treatment.

When you have someone new working in your home or providing personal services, such as cutting your loved one's hair, explaining her condition and the best way to deal with her can make the experience more pleasant for everyone.

> Earlene had been going to the same beauty shop for years, and the beautician and staff understood her condition and got along well with her. However, when a new receptionist was hired, no one remembered to tell her about Earlene.
>
> When she and her twin sister Carlene went for their monthly haircuts, Earlene stood at the counter and read aloud the captions on the posters that covered the walls.

53

The receptionist said, "Please have a seat. Your operator will be with you soon."

Earlene ignored her and continued to read aloud. The receptionist spoke a little louder, "There's another customer waiting behind you. Please sit down so she can step up to the counter."

At that, Earlene stopped reading and yelled, "Don't you scream at me! I'll stand here if I want to."

The receptionist spoke more forcefully. "Ma'am, please get out of the way."

By this time, Carlene, who had taken a seat as soon as they checked in, had returned to the desk. She motioned for the receptionist to move further down the counter and directed the customer who was standing behind Earlene in the same direction. The receptionist took care of the customer as Earlene continued to read from the posters on the wall, loud enough to be heard over the soft voices of the receptionist and customer.

The sisters were soon called—Earlene chatted with the stylist and her helper as if the incident at the front counter never occurred.

Carlene hurried back to the counter as soon as her hair was finished. She motioned to the receptionist, who stepped over to meet her saying, "I can't believe the rudeness of the woman you came in with!"

Carlene responded, "She's not rude—she's sick."

The receptionist said, "Sick! She looks perfectly healthy to me."

Carlene explained that her sister had AD and didn't understand that her behavior was rude. She continued, "If you had just ignored her and waited on the customer behind her, there would have been no harm done. You might have found her reading aloud annoying, but it didn't hurt anything. She only got loud enough to disturb others after you insisted she leave the counter. I'm sorry no one explained this to you in advance."

"Me, too," answered the receptionist. "Next time I come across a customer acting strangely, I'll try to handle it better."

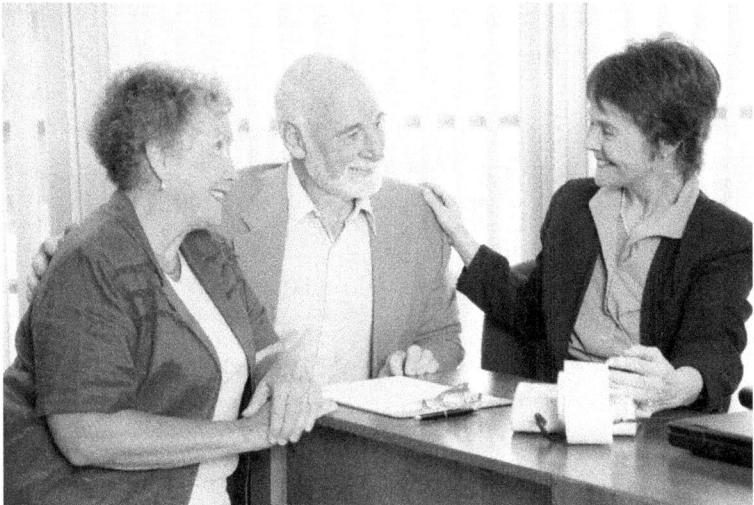

Enjoyable Things to Do

An Alzheimer's patient tends to be very restless. She may pace constantly or pick at the air. Keeping her busy may cut down on this and will also give her a sense of purpose. Tailor the activity to fit her ability and interests.

Activities should be kept short as the attention span of someone with AD is small. There is some evidence to suggest that persons with Alzheimer's, unlike people with other types of dementia, may have highs and lows when it comes to anxiety and energy. Most people with dementia peak and then the energy level falls. People with AD tend to have episodes of higher energy and then it falls or levels off, then it will rise and fall again. If you try to suppress this energy, it tends to return later at a higher level. It is better to try to use up this energy as it occurs.

- Make the focus of the activity enjoyment, not achievement. The end result is not important—participation is.
- The activity should focus on the abilities she maintains and not require the abilities she has lost.
- Allow her as much independence as possible.
- Be flexible and encouraging.
- Plan the activity when she is more alert. This will vary from person to person.
- Be sure instructions are simple. Do not overwhelm her with multiple step instructions.

Following is a list of activities she may enjoy. If she isn't interested in one, try another. Be innovative and come up with your own.

- Try to find activities that relate to her work or hobby experience. If she worked as a secretary, give her papers to sort and file into a box. If she was a homemaker, let her dust the furniture. If she loved to garden, give her a small garden area or a few houseplants that she can care for. Remember, the outcome doesn't matter. She may misfile the papers, leave dust on the furniture, or kill the plants with too much water. She is still doing something she enjoys and that gives her purpose and a feeling of being useful.
- Let her rake leaves in the front yard.
- Allow her to fold washcloths or towels and place them in a box. She will especially enjoy this if they are warm from the dryer.
- Give her a jar of buttons to sort (be sure she will not try to eat them).
- Encourage her to build with Legos or color a picture if she enjoys those activities.
- Take her to a garage sale. Things are usually inexpensive, so she can have the freedom to buy things, and you don't have to worry about the costs.
- Place Fruit Loops or Cheerios onto a string and hang them out for the birds to eat.
- Let her watch nature videos or movies from her younger days. She may understand these more easily than current programming.
- Go for a walk together.
- Let her perform tasks she may be familiar with in the kitchen—shucking corn, snapping peas, cleaning/sorting beans.
- Make no-bake dishes such as lemonade, pudding, fruit salad, and Rice Krispies treats.

- Bake cookies with her. This can be a good activity to do together—you can measure the ingredients, and she can help mix, roll, and cut out the cookies. She can even help decorate them.
- Have her assist with setting the table.
- Sing songs together. Even after having lost the ability to speak, AD patients often retain the ability to sing.

Romero had not spoken for nearly a year. He seemed to understand when given very simple instructions but did not respond when asked a question. He was in relatively good physical condition and was able to walk, participate in dressing, and feed himself. His loved ones often spoke to him, but they never got any response.

The family held a birthday party for one of Romero's grandchildren. The birthday cake was on the table, and everyone started to sing "cumpleaños felices." They were all amazed to hear Romero, loud and clear, singing every word.

While the cake was being cut, Romero started singing another song. He spent the next thirty minutes singing song after song and entertaining the whole family.

Once the party was over, Romero went back to his silence. The only time that he uttered a word was to sing, but he sang every time there was music. His family kept the radio on and he often sang along. They started taking him to church services, and he enjoyed singing his favorite hymns once again.

Nurture Spirituality

Often an Alzheimer's patient who has had a strong religious faith her entire life will remember things about her faith long after her memory has deteriorated.

Father Juan Garcia had been a Catholic priest for nearly fifty years. Although he had retired several years before his AD diagnosis, he carried a rosary and prayed throughout the day and attended Mass every Sunday. As his Alzheimer's progressed, he couldn't recognize family and friends, and he didn't know what day of the week it was—except on Sunday.

Somehow he always knew when it was time to go to Mass. His family didn't take him to church because they didn't know how he would act. When they could no longer care for him, they placed him in a nursing home.

The first Sunday in the nursing home, he got up saying it was time to go to Mass. The staff helped him dress and led him to the activity room, where a visiting priest was conducting services. Father Juan not only joined the congregational responses, but he said the entire Mass along with the priest.

That afternoon when his family came to visit, they were amazed to see him much calmer and happier than he had been in months. They regretted not taking Father Juan to services when he was still at home— they had no idea how much it meant to him.

Other residents of the facility also

benefitted from religious services, and the staff wanted to offer services every week rather than once a month as they did because of the availability of clergy. The administrator of the nursing home spoke to the bishop of the diocese about the situation, and the bishop authorized Father Juan to conduct Mass every week for the residents of the nursing home.

His family often attended the services to share this special time with Father Juan. Even residents of the facility who didn't seem to understand the service often came away calmer and more at peace than any other time.

If your loved one has a religious belief, she shouldn't be deprived of it now when she is deprived of so many other things. Perhaps she can't sit still long enough to attend services, but she might enjoy a few minutes of prayer and scripture with you. If she isn't interested in listening to words, she will likely enjoy religious music. As described in the story of Romero above, AD patients retain their memory for music much longer than their memory for words. She may not understand the words of a favorite hymn, but she can enjoy singing and experience the emotions the hymn evokes.

Don't forget your own spiritual health. Caring for your loved one can be very stressful, and you need not only physical and emotional support, but spiritual as well. You may have to adjust your spiritual practices to accommodate your caretaking, but you don't have to abandon them. If you can't leave your loved one to attend services at your church or synagogue, you may be able to find a televised or online service that you can watch. If the AD patient is willing to watch with you, you can benefit from the shared activity. If she will not watch with you, you can schedule the virtual service while your loved one is sleeping or otherwise occupied. You can find private devotional time for prayer, scripture reading, and meditation as well. If you are a religious believer, it is important for you to nurture your spiritual life.

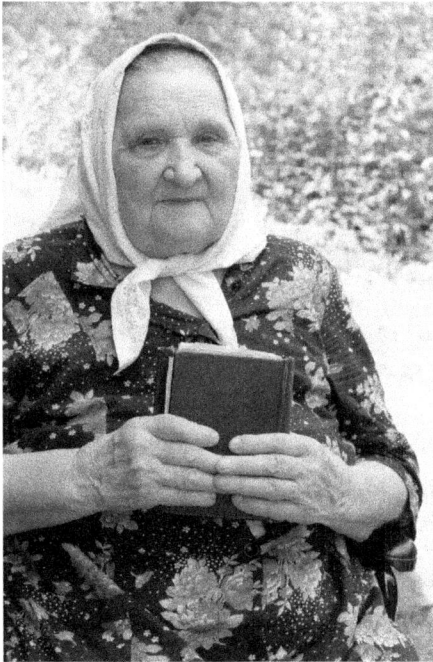

Laughter

Don't take yourself or your loved one too seriously. There will be plenty of opportunities to laugh. Take advantage of them and enjoy a good chuckle. Don't feel guilty about it. Just make sure that you are laughing at the situation and not at the person with Alzheimer's. They probably will not know what you are laughing about, but most often they will laugh along with you.

After my dad had been diagnosed with Alzheimer's, my mom wanted to take the opportunity to go to the Hill Country and see the trees changing colors. They took this trip every couple of years, and Mom wanted to go with Dad once more while she thought that he would still enjoy it. I was the designated driver, and I hate driving in *hills*. They seem like mountains to me.

Adding to my trepidation was the fact that it was raining. As we drove through the hills, my dad kept telling me how to drive. "Slow down;" "Don't get so close to the edge of the road;" "Be careful;" and on and on. I alternated between biting my tongue and assuring him that I would follow his advice. In an effort to help out, Mom kept trying to get Dad to be quiet, which actually made him and me more agitated.

When he kept telling me over and over that I was going to burn out my clutch (in an automatic), I replied, "Dad, I don't have a clutch."

He responded, "Well you shoulda listened to me. I told you that you were going to burn it out!"

I started laughing, and soon Dad and Mom both joined in. The pressure was released and Dad's apprehension lessened, as did mine. The rest of the trip was not worry free, but for a while we all got to enjoy a good laugh.

> *A cheerful heart*
> *is good medicine.*
> **Proverbs 17:22**

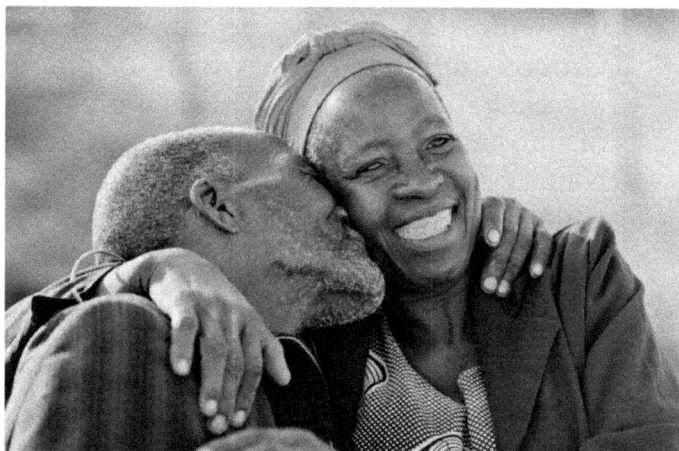

Taking care of yourself

Caregivers often neglect themselves, feeling that their wellbeing isn't as important as that of their loved ones. However, they cannot continue to provide good care for the AD patients if they let their own health and wellbeing suffer. To be able to continue to take good care of your loved one, you must take good care of yourself.

"When we truly care for ourselves, it becomes possible to care far more profoundly about other people. The more alert and sensitive we are to our own needs, the more loving and generous we can be toward others." ~ Eda LeShan

- Join an Alzheimer's support group. They have groups for spouses, families, and persons with AD. Some groups offer care for your loved one with AD while the meeting is being held. Groups are offered at a variety of times and places and even online. This is a great source of information and an excellent way to make contact with others who understand your situation.
- See your doctor regularly and follow his advice. You must maintain your own health to stand up to your caregiving challenges.
- Ask for help from family or friends who are familiar with Alzheimer's disease.
- If adult day care is available to you, use it to get a break.
- Get plenty of rest. This is possible only if you have help. See if a friend or family member can take him for a walk or to the park while you take a nap.

- Try arranging with another caregiver to keep her loved one occasionally, and she can return the favor. Someone who is dealing with the same issues as you are is more likely to be able to understand and handle your loved one. The two Alzheimer's patients may entertain each other, and while your loved one is with another caregiver, you can use the time to refresh yourself.
- Eat a healthy diet with plenty of fresh fruit and vegetables.
- Care for your spiritual health as well as your physical and emotional health.
- Even if the AD patient can't join in the laughter with you, enjoy a good laugh whenever you can.

Jay tended to get very agitated and angry when he got confused or forgot something. His wife Lana developed a routine that calmed him down.

"Do you remember that you love me?" she asked.

He said, "Yes."

"Do you remember that I love you?"

"Yes."

"Do you remember that Jesus died on the cross for your salvation?"

"Yes," he answered.

"Then you remember everything that is important. What you forget doesn't matter," Lana assured him.

This little ritual had been repeated effectively many times over months.

Then came the day that Jay was terribly confused about something. He became very agitated and angry.

"Do you remember that you love me?" Lana asked.

"Yes," he answered.

"Do you remember that I love you?"

"Yes."

"Do you remember that Jesus Christ died on the cross for your salvation?"

At that point, Jay turned to Lana with a look of total perplexity. "That was stupid!" he said.

At first, Lana was shocked and worried about Jay's apparent irreverence. Then she realized that from a human perspective, Jesus' sacrifice *was* stupid and made sense only from a spiritual perspective. Although she didn't laugh in front of Jay because he didn't realize what he had said, she has had many a good laugh with others over Jay's comment.

Now, when she wants to calm Jay down, she asks if he remembers that he loves her and she loves him. Then she asks, "Do you remember that God loves you, too?"

Remember Your Loved One Is Still in There Somewhere

The ravages of Alzheimer's disease are so devastating that it often seems that our loved one is no longer with us. We may feel like we're caring for the shell of the person we loved, but the essence of the one we loved is long gone.

The final days of my father's life convinced me that the dad I loved was still in there somewhere, even though we hadn't seen evidence of it for months. He had been born on the farm where he had lived his entire life except for his stint in the Army during World War II and those final months in the nursing home. He loved every inch of that ground, every animal, and every blade of grass. Our family wanted to honor his long-held and oft-repeated wish to die right there where he had been born and lived his life.

The nursing home called Mom early one morning and told her the end was near. Our family converged on the facility, which was more than an hour away from the homestead.

Dad was nonresponsive, as he had been for a long time, but the look in his eyes said a lot. The look of terror reminded us all of a trapped animal. Our hearts broke to see that fear, and we wondered if we were doing the right thing taking him on a journey he couldn't understand.

We secured Dad into a wheelchair and loaded him into my sister's wheelchair-fitted van. My brother-in-law drove the van, Mom and I were in my car, and my other sister followed in her car. All of us prayed all the way that Dad would live long enough to die at home.

When we arrived at the farmhouse, my teenage nephews and my brother-in-law struggled to get

Dad into the house and into bed. He acted like that trapped animal his eyes reminded us of, not wanting to venture into unknown territory. He could no longer see or hear, so he couldn't know where he was. We told him he was home, but we had no way of knowing if he understood.

Finally, we got him settled in bed. My parents' bedroom had windows all around the room, and we could see cows grazing in the pasture on a beautiful, sunny day. From the moment he arrived home, Dad was never left alone. My two sisters, my niece and two nephews, Mom, and I took turns sitting with him, holding his hand, and talking to him gently. We described what we saw outside the window. We told him how much we loved him. We made soothing sounds when we didn't have words to say.

Gradually that trapped-animal look disappeared from his eyes. His fearful, tense posture loosened. Amazingly, we saw a beautiful look of peace come across his face. He didn't respond in any way that we typically communicate with loved ones. He didn't look at us. He didn't speak. He didn't squeeze our hands. However, we could tell the essence of my father was still there. We saw his soul find peace at last.

The nursing home staff had told us Dad was within hours of death when we picked him up Tuesday morning, yet he was still with us Friday evening. My sister had read that sometimes people need permission to die. We didn't think Dad could hear or understand, but my sister decided to give him permission, anyway. She told him we all loved him and would miss him terribly, but if his work on earth was done, it was time for him to go home to the Lord. She assured him that he had lived a good life and had taken good care of all of us. She promised him we would take care of Mom and the farm. She reminded him again of how much we all loved him.

A few hours later he peacefully slipped away to heaven, where he'll never be touched by Alzheimer's again.

The disease had destroyed the last seven years of his life, but it didn't destroy the soul of the man we loved. Somewhere deep inside, my father was buried beneath the memory loss, the confusion, the agitation, and the loss of physical functions.

Even though it may not be apparent, remember the person you love is still there. Tell him often that you love him. Assure him that you want to care for him and that you consider it a privilege, not a burden.

You've probably been through many things in your relationship, and now you are on a new journey together. You still love each other. He may not be able to verbalize his love, but there will be moments that you feel it from a look or a touch. Those moments will give you the strength to face the tough challenges and make both of your lives as rich and full as possible.

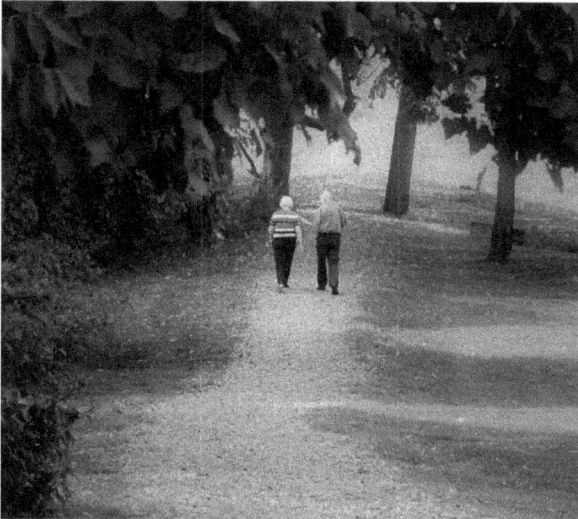

RESOURCES

Ageless Design—a resource for caregivers and professionals dealing with Alzheimer's disease: http://www.agelessdesign.com/

Alzheimer's Association—global voluntary health organization in Alzheimer care and support:
http://www.alz.org/
Alzheimer's Association
225 N. Michigan Ave., Fl. 17
Chicago, IL 60601-7633
(800) 272-3900
(312) 335-8700
Fax: (866) 699-1246

ALZBrain.org—information for caregivers and professionals from Dementia Education & Training Program through support from the Alabama Department of Mental Health and Mental Retardation and the Alabama state legislature: http://www.alzbrain.org/

Caring.com—information and support for caregivers for the elderly: http://www.caring.com

ElderCareOnline/Alzheimer's and Dementia Channel—resources for caregivers, including medical, financial, legal, and insurance information: http://www.ec-online.net/alzchannel.htm

ProHealth/Alzheimer's—current news on research and treatment, support groups, and more: http://www.prohealth.com/alzheimers/index.cfm

Nancy Nicholson

The 36-Hour Day: A Family Guide to Caring for People with Alzheimer Disease, Other Dementias, and Memory Loss in Later Life, 4th Edition. Nancy L. Mace, M.A., and Peter V. Rabins, M.D, M.P.H. The John Hopkins University Press, 2006.

Your state agency on aging—search online for "aging agency <state>" or "department of aging <state>"

Help! What Do I Do Now?

PERSONAL RESOURCES

Family and Friends

Name	Phone Number	Notes

Doctors

Name	Phone Number	Notes

Other Resources and Support

Name	Phone Number	Notes

Medications

Medicine	Dosage	Time Taken	Special Instructions (can crush, with food, etc.)

ABOUT THE AUTHOR

Nancy Nicholson traveled a circuitous route to her present position as a licensed social worker. She dropped out of college to go to work and spent years in a variety of careers, including nurse's aide, career counselor, and operations manager of an interior landscape company. When her father was diagnosed with Alzheimer's disease, she became one of several family caregivers. She watched her father deteriorate from a highly intelligent, strong, and independent man to a body lying in a nursing home bed, not recognizing anyone and unable to control his bodily functions. She also saw the toll the disease took on her mother, the primary caregiver, and the other family caregivers. What she saw made such an impact on her that she decided to return to college and devote her life to caring for the elderly, particularly patients with dementia. She graduated from Texas A&M International University with the degree Bachelor of Social Work and earned her license as a Licensed Bachelor Social Worker. For the past seven years, she has worked for a chain of nursing homes, first as a social worker in a facility and currently as a social services consultant, where one of her primary duties is training nursing home staff.

www.ingramcontent.com/pod-product-compliance
Lightning Source LLC
Chambersburg PA
CBHW070553030426
42337CB00016B/2473